I0407226

VITAMIN SOUP

A RECIPE FOR SOULFUL
NOURISHMENT FROM A TO Z

Sally Galloway
MME, CHHC, AADP

Natural Health Coach & Wellness Educator

VITAMIN SOUP

A RECIPE FOR SOULFUL

NOURISHMENT FROM A TO Z

Join our blog community, and get more goodies at *http://www.nutrition-counseling.com/spiritualfood*.

For information about special discounts on bulk purchases, write to: *soupgroup@vitaminsoupgroup.com*.

"I'LL HAVE THE SOUP"

Curl up in your favorite chair with *Vitamin Soup*! This brew offers a simple and delicious way to feed your mind, body, and spirit. I reach for these "vitamins" each morning for a nourishing start to my day.

Fabienne Frederickson, Client Attraction Mentor on Marketing and Mindset/Founder ClientAttraction.com

This is a must for everyone. My prescription is RX: *Vitamin Soup*, via the soul, daily. You will prosper abundantly in all areas of your life. Take <u>two</u> books, and pass this on to friends and family for their optimal well-being.

Alice Rodriguez Brockwell, ARNP Board Certified Family Nurse Practitioner

Vitamin Soup gives great examples/tips for obtaining a balance with food, exercise, and emotions. It's not all about the workout and calories consumed! Part of becoming healthy is striking a balance within your life. *Vitamin Soup* does a terrific job in helping you achieve that.

Deborah Cox, Certified Jazzercise Instructor

By nourishing the body with joy and reverence, we nourish the spark of life within the body. And when the body yields to disease and decay (which no amount of vegetables or vitamins can prevent), we are left with the knowledge that good nutrition is important but can take us only so far. The deeper nourishment that sustains heart and soul is what ultimately matters most.

Marc David, *Nourishing Wisdom*

INGREDIENT LIST

Acknowledgements

Thank you to all my clients, colleagues, and friends who contributed their soul-wisdom, generosity of spirit, authenticity, and ideas on how to supplement their own lives with these nourishing vitamins.

Thank you to my coaches, teachers, mentors, and facilitators, from grade school through my coaching and leadership training. Your lessons continue to feed me in many ways.

Thank you to the music directors and coaches who taught me to sing from my heart and who inspired me to live that way off stage, especially Janet Ashford, Kathy Carmody, Betty Clipman, Jim Copeland, Andre Thomas, and Robert Shaw.

Thank you to Tyler Kuethe for the lovely and whimsical illustrations. You remind us how easily we may find these vitamins if we simply open our eyes and hearts to look for them.

Thank you to Colette Joseph Blair for her friendship across the miles, insight, curious spirit, and editing skills which added tremendously to the delicious thoughts herein.

The biggest thank you of all goes to my wonderful husband, Doug Smith, my soul's supplement, who fills my vitamin soup bowl to overflowing each and every day.

Play With Your Food

Appetizers and Starters

First of all, let me share a little bit about my own journey to find s*oulful nourishment*. There are several major factors that impacted where I am today.

To begin with, I lost a very vital person in my life to cancer. At about the same time, I was exposed to massage therapy and started viewing health as something to be actively pursued rather than passively taken for granted. And finally, this book itself began when I heard a nutritional psychologist talk about our misplaced attempts to find real love and meaning through what we eat.

When he explained how we do not get sufficient quantities of Vitamin L, Love—especially from ourselves—I started thinking about other non-food things that nourish us as well. I also realized that where we are nourished, we may also be deficient. This started my search for ways to get more of these intangible but necessary things, just like you would decide to take a multivitamin or other supplement.

Some vitamins are easier to find than others.

When I was only 19, I lost my mother to colorectal cancer—she was only 41 years old. As you can imagine, in addition to the huge loss I felt, I was not quite ready to live life as a grown-up. I had so many questions to ask her: what to do about career choices, boys, cooking, and family issues. My primary advice-giver was gone, and I had no one to soothe the aches and growing pains of early adulthood. Talk about a deficiency of Vitamin L!

And yet, my mother's illness and untimely passing is what led me to the health, spiritual, and career path I am on today.

My mother passed away in October of my second year in college, while I was pursuing my first degree in music. The previous summer I had taken a class in basic massage therapy, so when I wasn't in music classes and recitals, I was teaching my classmates about eating better, preventing disease, managing stress, and having an active part in their overall wellness. I was always telling my classmates that wellness was "doing things to get even healthier when you are not sick, so that you can feel *great!*" I just wanted to share what I was learning about health with people I cared about so they could learn what it was too late to tell my mom.

A few years later, in my classes at massage school, I was exposed to the concept of the mind-body connection—that what we think (the mind) has an influence on our anatomy and physiology (the body). I also studied nutrition from both a physical and a spiritual perspective. I learned that what we put into our bodies and minds (what we eat and what we think) deeply affects our physical, mental, emotional, and spiritual health and well-being.

Although I did go on to finish my master's degree in music, my heart has always been in the health and wellness field. I felt I could (literally) touch so many more people and make a difference in a profound and lasting way.

While practicing massage therapy for a couple of decades and helping my clients discover their own mind-body connections, I was very fortunate to attend courses and conferences with Deepak Chopra and his team to learn about Ayurveda and natural health. I integrated this ancient knowledge into my healing practice and still apply its principles to my daily life.

To learn to teach through empowerment rather than lecturing, I was trained and certified as a life coach, a wellness coach, a group fitness instructor, and a holistic health coach and nutrition counselor.

However, this smorgasbord of certifications means virtually nothing without willing and motivated clients. Being able to witness some of my clients reduce or eliminate medications, reverse chronic health conditions, release fat permanently, start exciting new careers, and improve relationships with friends and family members, has been one of the greatest joys of my life!

My love of learning continues. I will always be a student of life, learning from my colleagues and my clients. I will forever be attending classes on anything that will help me better communicate my passion for helping others find nourishment, health, and wellness in every area of their lives.

And so, it is my greatest hope and desire to help *you* find all the nourishment and Vitamin L you so richly deserve and are entitled to—simply because *you are you* and *you exist*!

Serving Up Nourishment

Let's start by defining nourishment. Most people define nourishment as food (fats, proteins, and carbohydrates) and how these nutrients break down into vitamins and minerals. But real nourishment is far more than food!

Someone who is malnourished is portrayed as being underweight, having a bloated tummy, sunken, sad eyes, and looking very hungry. Rarely will you see a picture of a malnourished child smiling brightly for the camera.

On the other hand, when we see a picture of a person of healthy weight, with bright eyes, a good complexion, and looking fit, we think, "She is well-nourished."

Nourishment is so much more than what we eat, however. It is not solely about getting nutrients from food. *Soulful nourishment* is having meaningful things, activities, and people in your life who make you feel vibrant, happy, healthy, and alive. Proper nourishment brings you into a state of harmony with nature, others, and your own inner being.

You might be thinking of circumstances, like the end of a relationship or company layoff, when an entire pint of chocolate-chip ice cream seems extremely nourishing! No doubt that for a few minutes that ice cream does taste good. You probably do enjoy the smooth, creamy ice cream and the crunchy bits of chocolate. But at some point, the food we reach to for comfort—our comfort food—disappears, and our desire for true comfort remains unfulfilled.

When we talk about *soulful nourishment*, we are really talking about feeling good physically, mentally, emotionally, and spiritually. In this case, the ice cream may represent a hug or perhaps some reassuring words that would nourish you emotionally. The ice cream may simply be a more readily available source of comfort. Likewise, crunching on a bag of chips is a less volatile way of dealing with feelings of anger and disappointment. So we may eat chips rather than have a potentially difficult conversation we are putting off.

How many times have we all reached for food when we just wanted to feel better?

We all associate nourishment with food, but sometimes the food is only a substitute—and a temporary one at that—for what we really need and want.

I frequently ask clients to identify activities that they enjoy and make them feel good. You can do that too. Make a list of things you can do for yourself or with others instead of reaching for food. Create your own menu of the "comforts" or "vitamins" that you can quickly turn to when you are seeking solace or comfort.

Here are some ideas to get you started. Take a bubble bath. Go for a walk. Get a massage. Pet your cat. Call your mom, dad, or best friend. You will get to continue this later in the book.

Consuming Vitamin Soup

Vitamin Soup is as easy to follow as a well-worn recipe. You can easily find the "vitamins" you are looking for to increase the quality of your life just by flipping through these pages.

Multivitamins were created because food scientists understood that some vitamins work better when combined with other vitamins. *Vitamin Soup* also offers a broad-spectrum, multi-faceted approach to providing nourishment for you. When you combine the "vitamins" in this book, you can directly improve several areas of your life simultaneously.

Vitamin Soup nutrients all work in synergy. In other words, one vitamin by itself may provide temporary nourishment, but when you combine several of these vitamins, your results will be exponential.

As a holistic natural health "diva" (the music education had to show up *somewhere*) and an active food coach, I have heard as well as experienced first-hand, that the very things most people are missing from their lives are the "vitamins" in this book. When my clients work to increase these vitamins, they find:

- improved confidence and self-esteem
- deeper and stronger relationships
- strength and courage to be their "true self"
- new hobbies or a second (or third) career

And, as an added benefit—when they are more at peace with themselves, they often find it easier to nourish themselves physically and nutritionally—not out of obligation, peer pressure, or guilt, but out of self-love. This translates into weight loss, more energy to exercise or play, and a genuine desire to choose a healthier life!

After witnessing the nutritional transformations that occurred in my clients, my family, and me, I wanted to share this knowledge with you. It is my heartfelt hope that by reading this little book, you can heighten your awareness of how you can get more of these "vitamins" on your own, and thereby live a longer, happier, more nourished life.

A Heaping Helping of Vitamin Soup

It is not easy to change life-long habits and fill up some of the empty spots in our lives. It takes a bit of work, but hopefully this little book and the bite-sized homework activities will be easy and fun to accomplish. Here are some hints, but this is your book—so use them in whatever manner works best for you.

- Read about each vitamin and reflect on where it is or is not present in your life. Which vitamins are you missing?
- Look at each illustration for a moment. Close your eyes and imagine having more of that in your life. How do you feel? What emotions are you experiencing?
- Consider how you can obtain or increase that vitamin by playing with the activities listed.
- Enjoy yourself! Let this be fun and experimental. Approach these activities with curiosity and wonder. And feel free to "play with your food!"

Today's Special

I have created a special section to help you absorb and digest these vitamins more easily.

The **Supplements** section, located in the back of the book, includes guides, ideas, play sheets, and recipes for success. You can:

- create your very own **Nourishment Menu**
- enjoy a really fun day that both excites you and feeds your soul
- live your life in harmony with what is most important to you
- relax, reduce stress, and breathe deeply
- pamper and treat yourself
- ...and more!

Keep this little book beside your bed, in your bathroom, your kitchen, your work area, your car (or all of those). Go through it from front to back, over and over again, or open it at random and do whatever the "vitamin of the day" suggests.

You'll find the activities will get easier as you build the habit of self-nourishment. Space is provided for you to jot down notes about your experience so you can remember what works well for you.

Finally, please write to me through my website, or post a note on the blog so you can share your ideas, your personal recipes for success, and your good news with others. Let me know how your health is, where you are finding your own vitamins in your life, and what your favorite "vitamins" are.

http://www.nutrition-counseling.com/spiritualfood

As you experiment and play, you will find your own ways to supplement your life, and you will feel more nourished in mind, body, and spirit.

I wish you well.

> In health and harmony,
> Sally Galloway

> November 9, 2011

TAKE YOUR VITAMINS

Vitamin A: Attitude

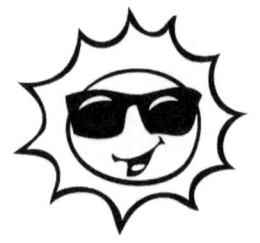

Your attitude determines how you interact with your surroundings and the people in them. The way you interpret events and activities is influenced by a positive or negative frame of mind. Since attitude is a choice—and yours alone—why not choose to be positive?

When you have a positive outlook and approach to life, you expect good things, and you look for good outcomes.

We attract what we focus on. Think about what you really want. Do you want to be healthier? Focus on healthy activities, foods, and people who make you feel good and strong.

Want to make more money? Place your attention on books, articles, and people who teach about making (and keeping) more money.

It all starts with you—so begin by being aware of your attitude.

Smile at someone today when you get on an elevator or when you pass someone on the street. Make eye contact and smile at someone. They may be surprised, but they'll probably smile back, and you'll both feel better!

Notes, ideas, results:

_____

_____

_____

_____

_____

Vitamin B: Books

Reading is an excellent tool for improving vocabulary, grammar, spelling, and intellect. Reading keeps your brain active and can give you a temporary break from stress.

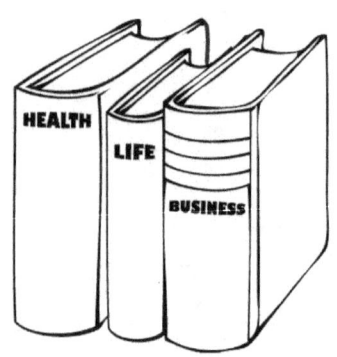

A good book can transport you to a mental vacation spot. Another can tell you about the real vacation spot. And yet a third can teach you the language or a skill to use when you visit that place.

If you look into the personal reading habits of the most successful people—those most sought after for their wisdom on life, health, and business—you will find they all read voraciously and have extensive book collections.

What's on your nightstand? What are you reading?

For some new ideas to feed your mind, check the Supplements for **Food for Thought**.

Consider expanding your physical library. Collect some books that address your personal interests and passions.

Mix it up: get some audio books to listen to while driving; curl up in a comfy chair with a cup of tea and a good book; hang out at a local café, and read on an electronic device.

Practice down time: indulge in enjoyment and relaxation with a love story or suspenseful mystery. Or expand your education: learn a foreign language; keep up with current events; become a brilliant conversationalist.

If you don't have the space or don't like collecting "stuff," get a library card and use it. There are many treasures to feed your brain in your local library.

Notes, ideas, results:

_____

_____

_____

_____

_____

Vitamin C: Color

Life is more interesting when we have color in it. Colors are imbued with different energies, and foods appear as different colors based on the nutrients they contain. Red, orange, and yellow foods contain *beta carotene*. Green foods contain *chlorophyll*. Blue and purple foods contain *anthocyanins*.

Red is associated with passion, strength, and energy.

Orange denotes inventiveness, creativity, and vibrancy.

Yellow is associated with a positive, sunny outlook and confidence.

Green represents health, healing, and happiness.

Blue helps to soothe and calm.

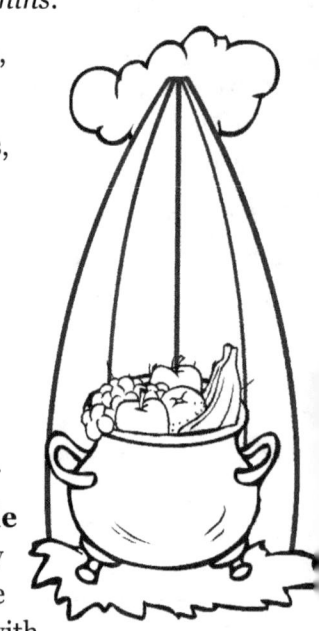

Indigo, violet, and purple are frequently seen on royalty and spiritual people—people who are comfortable with themselves and whom people like to follow.

What color do you want to be today?

Choose the energy you want more of, and put more of the color associated with that energy in your environment.

Strive to have more color around you, in your home or office, or on your plate. Here are some ideas:

Wear different colors. Paint a room. Buy some colorful flowers. Hang a new picture. Change your drapes or shower curtain. Have a different kind of salad a few days a week. Put as many colors on the plate as you can at each meal.

Notes, ideas, results:

_____

_____

_____

_____

_____

Vitamin D: Diversity

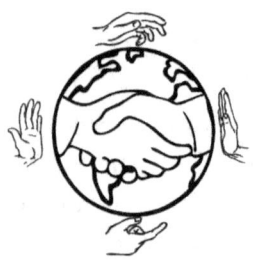

Ever heard, "Variety is the spice of life?" Well, Diversity is the pathway to variety.

Diversity as nourishment is about mixing it up. Enjoying variety in your relationships, the kinds of food you eat (not the same meals over and over again), and in the activities in which you engage, adds *spice* to your daily life.

Consciously choose to do something different from the way you usually do it. Do you always take a particular dish to a pot luck or dinner party? Do you always drive the same way to work?

Look for alternatives. Explore and embrace what they have to offer. Strive to make life interesting.

Today, take a different route to or on the way home from work. Eat a new food at a new restaurant or at home. Study a different culture or religion. Read a book or see a movie in a genre that is not your typical first choice.

Engage in conversation with someone you do not know well. Listen with an open mind and open heart. You may find you have more in common than you realized.

Exploring diversity has a way of bringing us closer together and revitalizing ourselves.

Notes, ideas, results:

_____

_____

_____

_____

_____

Vitamin E: Endorphins

Endorphins are our body's natural pain-killers. They are totally legal and—most of the time—fun to generate!

Endorphins are produced in the brain and are chemicals called neurotransmitters. They are released in many ways: when we exercise (runner's high), feel 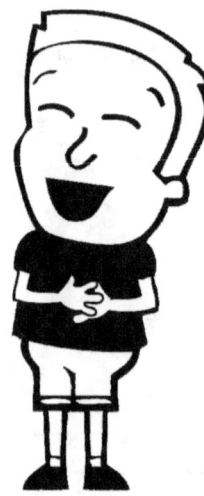 pain (bang an elbow), get excited (see an 80-yard catch and a touchdown), eat spicy food (wasabi rush), and when we experience orgasm (um...no real explanation needed).

If you just laughed or giggled, you released some endorphins!

Like the very strong pain-killers called opiates, endorphins create a feeling of well being; thus they are known as the body's natural morphine. They can produce an analgesic effect that supports our resolve to "get back in the game."

In the game of life, endorphins are a natural and nourishing reward for treating ourselves well.

There are numerous ways to release endorphins, pump up your immune system, and ultimately feel good.

Do something you like that makes time fly. Watch a funny movie, and laugh out loud. Take a long, brisk walk. Get a therapeutic massage. Order a hot and spicy dish. Enjoy a quickie or share a hug. Indulge in a few bites of high-quality chocolate. Immerse yourself in beautiful music or a sunset.

Notes, ideas, results:

_____

_____

_____

_____

_____

Vitamin F:
Friends and Family

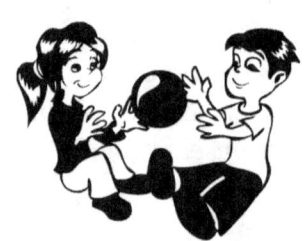

A strong connection with loved ones nourishes us on so many levels. Our hearts beat more strongly. Our confidence and self-esteem are boosted. We feel supported and encouraged by people who care for us. And we feel better about ourselves when we reach out and do something for those we love. We feel open, alive, and as if all things are indeed possible when we have close friends and family.

Feelings like anger, resentment, or guilt get in the way of feeling open and loving towards our family and friends. Harboring negative emotions can actually keep us from experiencing joy in the other parts of our lives.

By moving towards positive connections, we nourish ourselves and make room for healthier and happier relationships. Who can you reach out to today?

Have you ever gotten a little intuitive nudge to contact someone and didn't do it? And then you found out that person was ill—or worse? Take action to connect with those you value.

Make a date with a friend or a family member you haven't seen for a while. Write into your calendar an appointment to make that phone call you have been putting off. Enjoy time with a supportive and fun friend! Or, even better, be that supportive friend to someone else.

Notes, ideas, results:

_____

_____

_____

_____

_____

Vitamin G: Gratitude

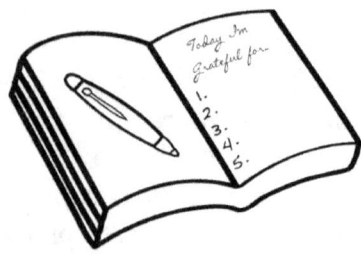

An "attitude of gratitude" keeps us focused on what we do have rather than on what we don't have.

Gratitude not only improves our mood and outlook, it makes it easier for us to notice when good things are coming into our lives so that we can take advantage of every opportunity.

Focusing your attention on what is good increases your ability to receive. This allows more things for which to be grateful to come into your life.

Purchase a pretty little journal that you can keep by your bed. Each evening before you lie down, write down five things you are grateful for. Recording thoughts in a journal helps our subconscious relax when we lay down to sleep. It also puts us in a more positive frame of mind and makes it easier to physically relax, go to sleep, and sleep more deeply. Good sleep leads to healthful restoration and healing on a cellular level.

BONUS: By keeping a Gratitude Journal, you are creating a reservoir of happiness and comfort that you can dip into when you experience a particularly rough day (it happens...). When you need help focusing on the good things in your life, just refer to your gratitude journal.

Notes, ideas, results:

_____

_____

_____

_____

_____

Vitamin H: Holism

A holistically healthy life is not just about being a certain weight or logging x minutes of exercise per week. Real holism looks at every system of the body and every area of your life. Holism considers how one part affects and interacts with the other parts.

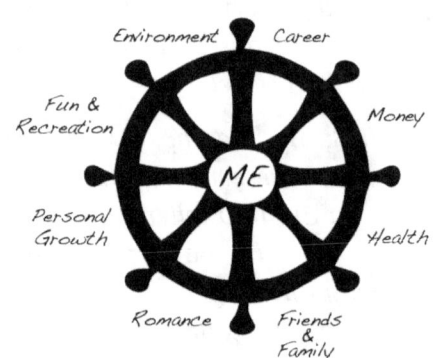

Holism also refers to the connection of your mind and body. Do you have an ailment, pain, or something that is just not going your way? Step back and look at your entire life and your whole body. What are you doing in one area that could be affecting another?

For example, is the clutter in your office affecting your ability to make clear-headed decisions?

Nourish yourself soulfully so that all aspects of your life are easier to swallow and digest.

Welcome to wellness.

On a piece of paper, draw a circle and divide it into eight "slices." Label each slice: Career, Money, Health/Fitness, Friends/Family, Romance, Personal Growth/Spirituality, Fun/Recreation, and Home Environment.

Rate your level of satisfaction in each area of your life on a scale of 1-10, with 10 being "great" and 1 being "something's gotta change." Notice how your level of satisfaction in one area affects your satisfaction in other areas.

If you were to do something different to increase your happiness in Health/Fitness, how would that impact and influence your happiness in Fun/Recreation?

Take action in one area and get ready for your whole life to get better!

*There is a copy of the **Wellness Wheel** in the Supplements section so you can check in with yourself regularly.*

Notes, ideas, results:

_____

_____

_____

_____

_____

Vitamin I: Integration

Integration is combining each area of your life so that you have enough energy and presence to enjoy and be successful in all of them. It's about combining your life's *have to's* with your *want to's*. You can increase the amount of happiness and joy in your life by pursuing a hobby or passion. The positive energy and excitement you generate from doing something you love can be tapped into and integrated into activities or events that don't get you so excited.

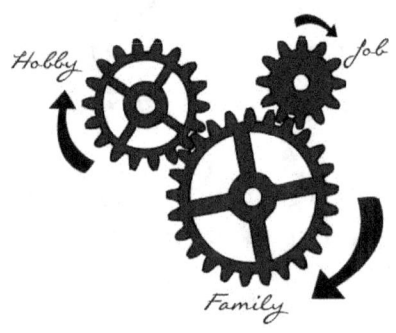

Integrated living keeps you moving forward towards accomplishing your life's goals and dreams. It helps you create a full life that's both deeply satisfying and nourishing.

Make a list of the things you would do if time and money weren't a factor. Choose just one thing, or even a small aspect of that thing, from your list. As you go through your daily activities, try to integrate that one thing into your life in some way.

For example, maybe singing is a passion for you, but you cannot pursue it as a career. Start your day singing in the shower, or put a favorite CD in your car, and give yourself a mini-recital on the way to work. It'll brighten your mood, and the people in the cars around you will smile just because they will recognize you are having a good time! Integrate what you love to do into what you need to do.

Notes, ideas, results:

_____
_____
_____
_____
_____

Vitamin J: Juiciness

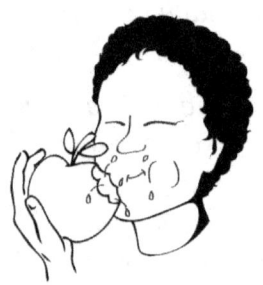

Which sounds like more fun: "Have a nice day!" or "Have a juicy day!" Oh, yeah. Definitely *juicy*.

What pops into your mind? What makes you *really* happy?

When you create your to-do list for the day or week, what do you always do first (regardless of its priority)? Conversely, look at what you avoid doing—no matter how urgent or high on your list it is.

What do you end up focusing on or choosing to do even if it is not among your top priorities?

Which parts of your life excite and energize you? Washing the dishes? Walking your dog? Reading a novel? Writing a blog post?

What in your life is juiciest? Enjoy more of that!

What in the previous list (or your own list) feels exciting, increases your energy, and makes you smile just thinking about it? Well, do that, and love every second of it. You can then transfer that "juice" to something else on your to-do list with more energy and enthusiasm to get it done.

Do something juicy every day. You deserve it!

Look for your **Have a Juicy Day** *to-do list in the Supplements section.*

Slurp!

Notes, ideas, results:

_____

_____

_____

_____

_____

Vitamin K: Kisses

Did you know that the lips have thousands of nerve endings and are one of the most sensitive areas of the body?

The nerve endings there are more densely packed than anywhere else, and the skin on the lips is thinner than other areas on the body (only 3-5 cells deep). This allows us to feel even the slightest touch with more acuity, setting off a torrent of activity in the brain.

According to WebMD, the act of kissing has some pretty interesting health benefits. Exchanging big wet ones can burn calories (do not confuse this with a good cardio workout, but you never know what passionate kissing can lead to...), and you will tone your 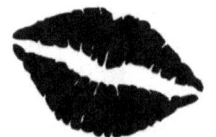 facial muscles, keeping you looking younger and happier. And feeling younger and happier is nourishing for your soul.

Just for fun, see how many kisses you can collect during a day or a week. Get them from your lover, your kids, your pets, your friends.

If you are in a committed, romantic relationship, one of the best ways to reconnect with your loved one, help improve communication, relax, and release endorphins at the end of the day is a 10- to 20-second kiss. Try it!

Notes, ideas, results:

_____

_____

_____

_____

_____

Vitamin L: Love

Ahh, Love...
L'amour. Liebe. Amor.
Szeretet. Amore.

Cue the violins!

No matter in what language we say it, we all want it. It feels great to receive, and even better to give. Love comes in many forms, depths, and degrees of intimacy. Love can cheer, console, support, encourage, and nourish us.

Think about the love that goes into the food we prepare for ourselves and for our loved ones. There is a reason why "mom's home cooking" always rates so high. She makes it with love. Love's the secret ingredient that is acquired in bulk and can be mixed into anything we prepare.

Even when you can't control who makes your food, you can sprinkle a little love or a blessing over the food you are about to consume. Being thankful is a form of love—and it makes everything taste better!

Before you quickly ingest your next meal, take a few minutes to think about its origins. Give thanks and love to all who were involved in getting it to you: the growers, the pickers, the sellers, the buyers, the people who pay you so you can purchase it, and the people who prepared it for you (even if that person is you).

If you are having a bad day, do something nice for someone else. You don't even have to know the person. Just spread a little sunshine. Put a quarter in a meter that's about to expire. Pay the toll for the car in back of you. Take an extra 30 seconds and hold the door for someone approaching slowly. Next time you cook for someone, consciously add "love" as an ingredient. It just might "spice up" your love life!

Notes, ideas, results:

_____

_____

_____

_____

_____

Vitamin M: Money

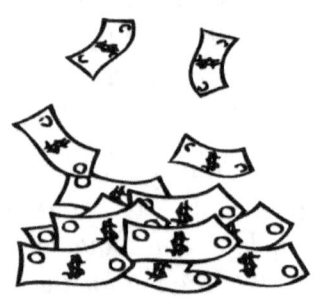

Whoa! Money? If you are thinking that you can't be focused on money while living a more spiritual life, you are probably not alone; but money is a necessary nutrient in our lives and is not inherently bad.

Vitamin M could also be meditation or music or motivation—we all benefit from those, too. But money is a key element for getting what we want and need from life—like clothes and a place to live!

Here is a question for you: Is it easier for you to have the life you want if you have money or if you don't? Some level of financial security allows us to serve others, pay the mortgage, take the kids on a vacation, treat ourselves to luxuries like pedicures, and maybe even take some time off to write a book.

Having enough money enables us to feed our bodies with fruits and vegetables and feed our souls with the types of vitamins in this book!

You can feel wealthier by keeping a clean, crisp $50 or $100 bill in your wallet. Don't spend it. Just keep it there. When you see it as you go to pay for something, say to yourself, "there is always enough." Seeing that you have more creates a feeling of abundance and starts to build a healthier relationship with money.

The well-known adage, "Ask and you shall receive," has been updated in today's spiritual literature. "Give and you shall receive" is a more effective—and more rewarding—way to accumulate both material and spiritual wealth.

If you do not give to a charity, tithe to a church or a religious organization, or volunteer at some level, add one of these things to your financial goals for the upcoming year. If you already give, where can you increase your contribution?

Notes, ideas, results:

_____

_____

_____

_____

_____

Vitamin N: Nature

"Go take a hike!" is good advice for nourishing our mind, body, and spirit. We are created of the same "stuff" that also makes up the great outdoors: water, air, space, fire, and earth.

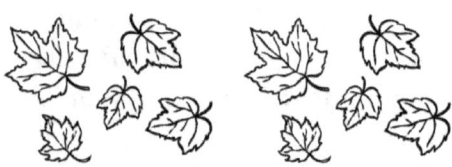

Look skyward to see the twinkle of a million stars, and experience the vastness of space. Watch the leaves spin in circles, and observe the power of wind. Feel the comfort of a campfire, even as it consumes and transforms its own fuel. Observe the relentless ocean waves, and witness the power of water. Take in the majesty and power of the mountains, and sense the stability of our earth.

While some people enjoy the beach and warmer climes, others prefer the country, mountains, or a cold-weather adventure. No matter what our individual preferences are, when we "get back to nature," we all share feelings of being rested, rejuvenated, and restored. Go outside, and get close to nature; harmonize with the elements from which you are made.

How do you get close to nature? Where do you see yourself harmonizing with the elements? Do you see aspects of yourself in the sway of the trees, the boundlessness of the sky, the powerful ocean, a crackling fire, the steadfastness of mountains?

To regain life balance and calm your mind, body, and spirit, step outside and put your feet in the grass, wiggle your toes in the sand, or dig your fingers into the dirt.

If you seek restoration and rejuvenation, hike in the mountains, play in the ocean, walk along the beach, stroll through a park and listen to the birds. Or just sit on the porch and watch the sunset in appreciative silence.

Notes, ideas, results:

_____

_____

_____

_____

_____

Vitamin O: Oxygen

Oxygen is the stuff we use to breathe in the fullness of life. In our hurry-up, get-it-done world, we are reluctant to stop and breathe deeply. We might miss a call, an email, a text—we can't slow down too much or we may never finish our errands! Yikes!

STOP. Can you feel your breath getting high in your chest, shallow, and quick just imagining your to-do list and all the rushing around you need to do? How does it feel when you grab some food and throw it down while you are on the run? Have you ever realized that you had eaten a meal but didn't even remember what it was or what it tasted like? Are you hungry again soon afterwards?

There is a very easy and effective way to move from fast-paced and nutrient-poor "feeding" to purposeful, healthy, and *full-filling* nourishment. In about a minute, you can increase your concentration, think more clearly, and even improve your digestive effectiveness. Getting more nutrients and satisfaction from your food and life is as easy as taking a deep breath!

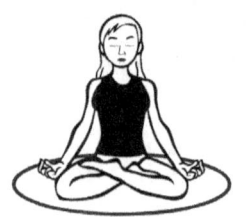

Sit with your spine straight, head floating, and your feet flat on the floor. Take a deep breath in through your nose, feeling your belly expand and the coolness of your breath passing through your nostrils and into your lungs. Exhale slowly and completely through your mouth, allowing your belly and ribs to relax and soften. Repeat for 5-10 breaths.

If you find yourself rushing to eat, put your fork down, close your eyes, and take three slow, deep breaths. Breathing deeply shifts your body from a stress response to a relaxation response—the one that supports digestion.

*Do this anytime you need to relax. It will feed you on many levels. Other ways to **Breathe—for Life** are in the Supplements.*

Bon appetit!

Notes, ideas, results:

_____

_____

_____

_____

_____

Vitamin P: Pleasure

The human body is wired to move toward pleasure and away from pain. Maybe that is the secret to our survival. People live longer, healthier, and certainly happier lives, when they pursue pleasure consciously and with purpose.

What brings you true pleasure and fills your very soul? Make a list of the things in your life that you love; then make the conscious decision to experience more of them. Remember: it is much easier to receive pleasure from someone and something else when you know how to obtain pleasure for yourself.

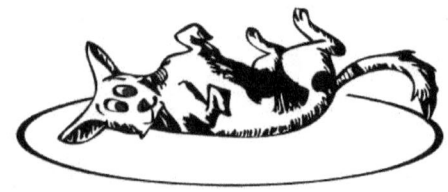

To make this type of pleasure a potent supplement, increase what gives you, and only you, pleasure. Picture yourself as a dog or a cat. What makes you wag your tail? What makes you purr?

Make it your priority to discover your body, to engage your senses, to notice what pleases you, causes you to smile, and makes you feel good. This is nourishment at its deepest, most intimate, and most personal level.

Think about the people in your life. Who do you truly love being around?

*What kinds of activities bring you intense and immense pleasure? Strive to have more of those activities in your life. Your Supplements section has a two-part **Pleasure Play List** for your enjoyment.*

Notes, ideas, results:

_____

_____

_____

_____

_____

Vitamin Q: Quality

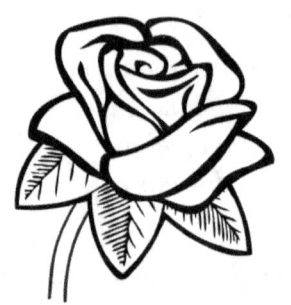

When we are small, we all have big dreams—to become an astronaut, the President of the United States, a tennis all-star, a millionaire, the perfect mate with a beautiful family.

As we go through life, we inevitably experience someone saying "no." We experience things that don't turn out exactly as we hoped. When disappointment happens often enough, the common response is to reduce the size of our dreams! Our comfort zone gets a little smaller, and we stop reaching for the big prizes we used to think so easily within our grasp.

Please don't settle! Go for what you want!

Yes, it probably will feel uncomfortable and scary, but that just means you are on the edge of what you know, and you are about to venture into the territory of your dreams. Give yourself the freedom of uncertainty, and enjoy the unfolding mystery of the deepest and most long-lasting personal growth possible. You are worth it!

Make a list of the stuff you want—what you really want. Look outside of your comfort zone and habits. Dream big—really big!

Make another list of things you want to do. Go wild. Have travel in mind? Where to? Want to start another career? Or maybe retire soon?

Finally, who do you want to be? What legacy do you want to leave when you leave this world? How do you want to be remembered?

What is your vision for your life? Commit to getting what you want. Believe it is possible and that you are worthy of your dreams. Put your full attention to BE-ing a high-quality person. Set goals, and take the action necessary to reach those goals.

Your **Be, Do, Have List** *is in the Supplements section. Think like a child again!*

Notes, ideas, results:

_____

_____

_____

_____

_____

Vitamin R: Relaxation

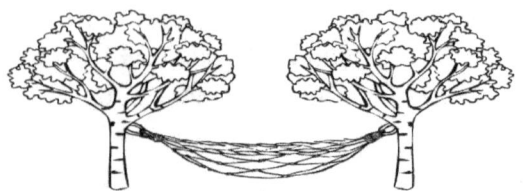

In my practice, I meet some extremely successful and very fast-moving clients. When they describe their lifestyles and daily schedules, I get tired just listening!

When I ask these high-achievers what they do for relaxation, they usually reply with "exercise," "cleaning the house," or "gardening."

While these activities can indeed be relaxing at times, "doing" is not true relaxation. Soulful relaxation is the rejuvenation and restoration that comes from...wait for it...doing *nothing*. Yes, sitting or lying down, and just *BE*-ing still.

I am not saying you should become a lump on the couch, but in order to hear and acknowledge the small voices that feed your creativity and passion, you must balance activity with relaxation. When your brain is so busy and noisy, the soft sounds of your true self cannot get through. Don't miss out on what your heart is trying to tell you!

We are human BE-ings; not human DO-ings, but if you feel the urge to "do" something, DO this:

- *Set a timer for 5 minutes.*
- *Sit down with your back straight, feet on the floor, hands in your lap.*
- *Close your eyes.*
- *Silently mouth the word "so" on your inhale. Silently mouth the word "hum" on your exhale. Repeat until the timer goes off.*

Listen to your inner-most self—what is your heart trying to tell YOU?

If you feel more relaxed or even more rejuvenated, congratulations!

If you fell asleep, you have not done anything wrong—it just means you're sleepy and didn't know it!

Relax and Restore *is in Supplements.*

Notes, ideas, results:

_____

_____

_____

_____

_____

Vitamin S: Simplicity

Do you find that life is often just too complex? As a culture, we are desperately looking for ways to make life easier and simpler.

Here is what we *think* we are seeking:

- *feng shui* consultants and personal organizers to simplify living and work spaces
- personal chefs to come into our homes to prepare a day's or a week's worth of food for us
- 30-minute meals with a few ingredients that we can pronounce and easily find
- quick exercises that we can work in to the nooks and crannies of our day
- social networks that let us keep in touch with multitudes of people without too much effort

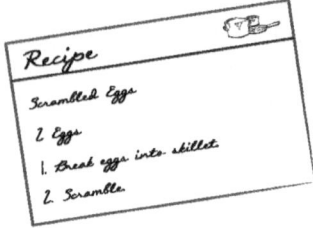

Even just reading this list can be overwhelming when you already have too much on your plate. And did you notice that most of what we are searching for are just tools that enable a more hectic pace? While there is certainly value to be gotten from all the things on the list, why not strive to change your pace? Then, instead of needing all the tools to get through life, you can enjoy them.

To simplify your life, start with ONE thing you will focus on that will create space in your life.

Clean out a drawer or closet. Take some clothing to a local charity. Throw away old spices you haven't used in a few months.

You may find that the mere act of clearing out and simplifying your surroundings will build momentum, creating space and simplicity in ways you cannot yet imagine.

Let's keep it simple: just take the first step.

Notes, ideas, results:

_____

_____

_____

_____

_____

Vitamin T: Time

Did you know that there is a way of eating called the *Slow Food* movement? *Slow Food* is characterized by taking ample time to prepare a meal of local, organic foods. It is a method of dining slowly and luxuriously, preferably with friends and family. *Slow Food* is also a wonderful way to nourish yourself when dining alone.

Several things happen when you slow down. You make the meal an event—something to be savored, celebrated, and enjoyed. You deepen your relationships and strengthen your bonds. Your full attention is on the loving and mindful preparation and presentation of the food—food made with love and the conscious intention of nourishing the total person.

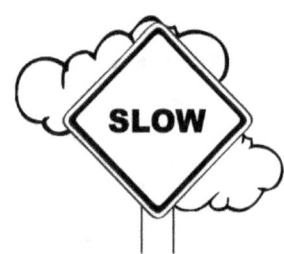

When you slow down, your focus is on *full-fillment*, not on feeling full. You may find you are eating less, reducing your caloric intake, and even shedding a few pounds! And your digestive system can fully assimilate the food in a relaxed and natural way, yielding greater nutrients and more nourishment.

You can slow down and experiment with the Slow Food method anytime. You simply have to choose to do it and plan for it—because it is not typical in our culture to allow more than 30-60 minutes from start to finish for any meal.

Whether just for yourself, or with friends or family, plan a meal, shop deliberately, and prepare the cooking and eating space. Set the table with the "good china," flowers, and candles. Play some music, and take your time. Utilize all of your senses with every bite—see the colors, smell the food, feel the textures, hear the crunch, and taste the variety of flavors.

En-JOY!

Notes, ideas, results:

_____

_____

_____

_____

_____

Vitamin U: Understanding

In terms of soulful nourishment, we are fed at a deeper level when we put our need to be heard and to be seen aside, and really listen to the person sitting across from us.

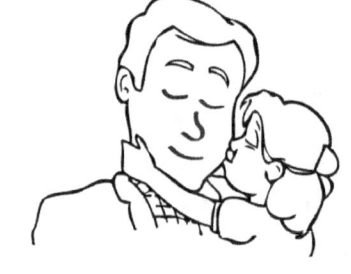

One of the "seven habits" that author Steven Covey found in very successful people, is that they *seek first to understand, and then to be understood.* This same habit of active listening and compassionate understanding is likely found among the most well-nourished people we know.

Have you ever heard a teacher or a parent say, "We have two ears and one mouth"? Our very anatomy, not to mention a lot of "grown-ups," just might be trying to tell us something important!

Listen first with an open heart and open mind. Have you ever "jumped in" before someone was done talking because you feared you wouldn't get a chance to say what you wanted to say? Or you "knew" what they were going to say and just wanted to get your time to talk—or correct them? This comes from not being fully present for the other person in your conversation.

When you listen first, with an open heart and a genuine desire to understand, you will then have the presence and the capacity to say what you need to say. And they will hear you better, too.

Breathe, and then speak from your heart. The right words will come.

Notes, ideas, results:

_____

_____

_____

_____

_____

Vitamin V: Vibrancy

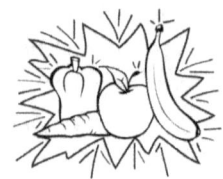

Picture a bowl of applesauce. Now picture a fresh apple. Which is more vibrant? The apple, right? Of course!

Why? Because it is vibrating with life energy. It is in a state that is close to its source—the tree, water, rain, and sun. Once it has been cut and processed, the connection to its source is harder to discern.

That is how it with us, too. We vibrate, pulse, dance, shimmer, and flow with life when our energy is closer to our source. Vibrating in harmony with our source—being in resonance—is a healthy, exciting, powerful way to nourish our souls.

When we connect to our source, we feel resonance with those around us as well—because in reality we are all connected by the same energy. We can feel when we are living our lives in harmonic resonance with our values and our life purpose. Barriers to success and differences between people dissolve. We feel more alive and confident—we vibrate with excitement about life, with possibility and power—when we stay true to who we are.

What are the 10 values that are most important to you? Values are not about right and wrong. They are aspects or qualities that you cannot live without. See **Values for Vibrancy** *in Supplements for more ideas.*

Here are some examples, but use your own words:

Connection	*Courage*
Health	*Humor*
Love	*Adventure*

Take a good look at your list. Are you living your life in harmony with your values? Are you vibrating in resonance with what is most important to you in your life?

Choose the value that has the highest vibration for you and makes you feel most connected to your source. Live from there today, and notice how vibrant your life is.

Notes, ideas, results:

_____

_____

_____

_____

_____

Vitamin W: Water

It is pretty common knowledge that water promotes weight loss, digestive health, skin health, and gives us a vibrant glow.

But the nourishment that you can get from water is not limited to its internal health benefits.

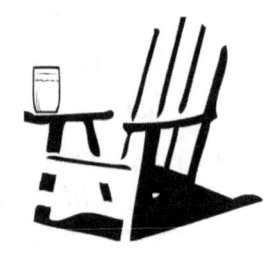

Many people feel refreshed by simply looking at a body of water. It has a calming effect on the mind, and just thinking about going to the beach, taking a cruise, or walking along the seashore makes people want to take a deep, cleansing breath!

The sound of water itself is soothing. It is no wonder that the sound of babbling brooks, ocean waves, and rain showers are frequently featured on "relaxation CDs."

And, finally, the mere touch of water is luxurious when you feel the gentle rain on your skin, are submersed in a warm bath with an essential oil like lavender, or are floating dreamily on a clear, salt-water sea.

Find some pictures of water that inspire you. Go to the ocean, a lake, or visit a waterfall. Enjoy a day at a water park, or go swimming.

To aid in relaxation, play a CD that features the sounds of water.

Upon waking, indulge in a glass of hot water with fresh lemon juice. This cleanses the liver and flushes toxins.

If you feel thirsty or are dehydrated, take sips of water every 15 minutes instead of downing a full glass of water. Just like a thirsty plant, that water will go right through you, so take your time to replenish yourself. Focus on nourishing your body's tissues with smaller amounts of water over time so you can get and stay fully hydrated.

Notes, ideas, results:

_____

_____

_____

_____

_____

Vitamin X: Xeriscape

Xeri-*what*? If this term is new to you, don't worry. It will not take long before you start hearing more about this concept of being respectful to the earth and nourishing the planet on which we live.

Xeriscaping (pronounced "zehr-i-scaping") comes from the Greek word for "dry" (*xeros*) and "landscaping." This concept is credited to employees of Denver Water in Denver, Colorado and has been around for about 30 years. Xeriscapes originally were focused on landscaping or gardening methods that minimized the use of water, but the concept has already expanded.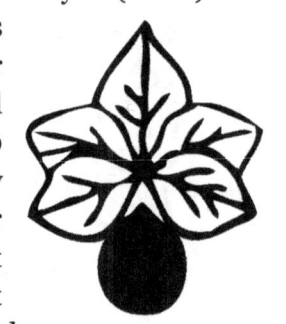

Xeriscapes also use native plants that are appropriate to the climate where they are planted. This helps to reduce the consumption of imported or ground water. "Planting local" is a way of practicing conservation and preservation.

Nourish the earth. Give something back.

Want to get back to nature? Here are some ways you can nourish the ground you walk on, keep your lawn green, and maybe even get more "green" back into your pocket:

- *Create a rock garden.*
- *Water your lawn with a hose, not a sprinkler—this reduces misting and evaporation.*
- *Replace a high-water-consumption area of your lawn with a relaxing place to sit. Decorate with stones, mulch, and a park bench.*
- *Visit your local nursery and ask about xeriscaping. They will help you choose native stones and the drought-resistant plants that are more likely to thrive in your area.*

Notes, ideas, results:

_____

_____

_____

_____

_____

Vitamin Y: Yes!

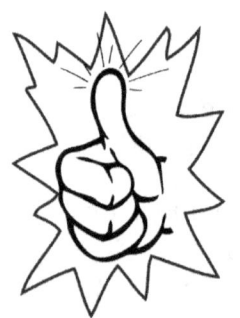

Saying "Yes!" is a signal to the Universe (and also to your subconscious) that the green light is on and that you are open to receiving good things into your life. Saying "Yes!" increases the flow of energy toward creating what you want.

Say the word "Yes!" either out loud or to yourself, with enthusiasm and power. Notice how your body feels.

Now say the word, "No!" with just as much enthusiasm and power. How does your body feel now? Do you feel a shift in your mood? Your breath? Your posture?

"Yes!" has more positive "vibes" and therefore creates a positive, hopeful shift in your feelings.

"No" creates resistance and makes it harder for you to access creative energy.

Say "Yes!" to nourishing and nurturing yourself. Affirm who you are in your heart and what you want for your life.

Say "Yes!" to opportunities that come up in your life. When you are nudged to take action, take it. When you set your sights on a change you want to make and a person or idea comes to you that could make that possible, say, "Yes!"

In addition, because "Yes!" feels better than "No," get your mind to a place of "Yes!" as soon as possible when faced with a situation that is painful or contrary to what you expected. By getting yourself to a place of acceptance, you are able to assimilate the change, or reality and truth of your situation in a much more peaceful way than if you fight or resist.

Go for it and go forward.

Notes, ideas, results:

_____
_____
_____
_____
_____

Vitamin Z:
Zest for Life

Zest for Life encompasses all of the preceding vitamins and nutrients. It is actually the enzyme, or catalyst, that makes digestion and assimilation of all these vitamins possible.

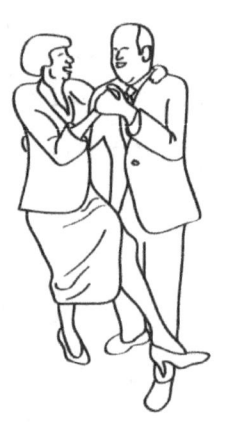

Without Zest for Life, you cannot fully appreciate the sumptuousness of a kiss, the vibrant colors of a rainbow (either in the sky or on your plate), or the simple joy of accomplishing even the most basic of tasks.

When you fully appreciate your existence and make the choice to be happy every day, no matter what curves life throws at you, you turn every setback into an opportunity to learn something new, and every success into a stepping stone towards something even more wonderful.

Practice being happy. Choose words that are uplifting, encouraging, and positive. (This includes the words you say to yourself).

*The **Play List (Part 2)** in Supplements is all about words.*

Focus joyfully on the things you want, who you want to be, and what you want to do. Then you can take appropriate action to attain those things. Spend time with people who are joyful.

When you discover something that does not work for you—celebrate it! Then you are free to focus on the things that do work in your life.

And most importantly, remember to be completely present. NOW is the time for you to fully experience every minute of your rich and delicious life!

Notes, ideas, results:

_____

_____

_____

_____

_____

THANKS, COME AGAIN!

Well, you did it! You got through an entire menu of ideas, some of which might have been quite an adventure for you.

As a holistic health coach and not a registered dietician, I am a big advocate of experimentation rather than prescribed "do it this way" food plans, especially when it comes to playing with your food—and with what truly feeds your mind and soul. I don't believe there is one right way to live healthfully. A simple "calories in, calories out" formula just *does not work*. Every *body* is different. You have probably discovered for yourself that there is more to health and happiness than diet and exercise.

To be truly nourished, you need to discover what works best for you, your lifestyle, your likes and dislikes, and your wellness goals.

So what was on *your* list of vitamins? Which ones did you notice you already "take" as part of your daily regimen? And in which vitamins are you deficient? Which ideas and activities are you going to implement in order to make up for your deficiencies?

What are the vitamins that show up in your life that are different from those in this particular batch of soup?

You could positively influence your friends and family by being their "personal nourishment chef" and sharing this information with all of them—make your own multi-vitamin soup!

Create your own list of soulful vitamins on **My Nourishment Menu** in the Supplements. Then be sure to share your customized vitamin list on my blog, *http://www.nutrition-counseling.com/spiritualfood*. Finally, put the list on your refrigerator so you remember to take your vitamins every day!

Scribbles, Nibbles, and Nuggets of Wisdom

_____

_____

_____

_____

_____

_____

_____

_____

_____

_____

_____

_____

_____

_____

_____

_____

_____

_____

_____

_____

_____

_____

_____

Supplements

PERSONALIZED NUTRITION

My Nourishment Menu

What nourishes my body, feeds my mind, and
supplements my soul:

_____

_____

_____

_____

_____

_____

_____

_____

_____

_____

_____

_____

_____

_____

_____

_____

Vitamin Guides

Be, Do, Have Wish List

Put your feet on the floor, place your hands in your lap and take three deep breaths, letting your body relax completely.

Take your mind back to when you were 7 or 8 years old. Imagine the house you grew up in, the school you went to. See yourself on the playground with your friends, talking about all the things you will do when you grow up, what you will be, and all the nice things you will have.

Now imagine that you are in your early 20's, just beginning your career, and dreaming about all the things possible for you. You have no limitations on your time, and you are making all the money you need. Whatever you choose for your life is possible. What do you want to do? How do you want to spend your time?

5 things I want to do

1.

2.

3.

4.

5.

Now look down beside you. There is a copy of the infinite *Catalog of the Universe,* and you have a gift certificate! Browse through and choose any five things you want. What will you get? What kind of house would you like to have? What will be in the house? What kind of car is in the driveway? What do you want to show your friends and family?

5 things I want to have

1.

2.

3.

4.

5.

Now see yourself quite a bit older, knowing that you are coming to the end of your full and happy life. What is the legacy you are leaving behind? How will people remember you? What have you accomplished?

5 things I want to be

1.

2.

3.

4.

5.

Breathe—for Life

Breath is the connection between the brain and the body. How we breathe sends a signal from the brain to the body to indicate our state of health—emotionally and physically.

Feel the difference between shallow and deep breathing by placing one hand on your chest, and one on your tummy.

Make your chest rise and fall. Feel your shoulders moving too? This activates the sympathetic nervous system, known as the "fight or flight" response.

Shallow breathing results when we are under stress.

Now take your focus lower and make your tummy rise and fall. This activates the parasympathetic nervous system, known as the "feed and breed" response.

Deep breathing induces relaxation, allows access to emotions, and improves digestion.

The following breathing techniques, used properly, reduce stress and activate a relaxation response. Go at your own pace and always start with several natural breaths, then move into these breathing practices.

To Calm the Mind (Three-part Breath)

If you are new to diaphragmatic breathing, it is nice to start by lying on your back so you can feel the full movement of the breath in the body.

Inhale deeply—fill the belly up like a balloon, let the breath travel up to expand the rib cage, and then draw it into the upper chest. Exhale—let the breath go from the upper chest, then from the rib cage, and finally from the belly, drawing the navel back toward the spine. Repeat 3-5 times. Then relax. Bliss!

To Cool Down (Shitali Breath)

Stick your tongue out and roll it like a tube (if you can). Bring the lips close around the tongue.

Breathe in deeply through the mouth. You will hear a hissing sound ("sssssss").

Exhale slowly through the nose.

Repeat 5-10 times until you feel the coolness spreading in your body.

To Energize (Ujjayi or "Ocean Breath")

Inhale through your nose.

On the exhale, gently close the space in the back of your throat between the roof of your mouth and the back of the tongue. You will hear a "whooshing" sound, like the ocean. Try to do this on the exhale and the inhale for maximum effect.

Food for Thought

Here are some of my favorite books to nourish mind, body, and spirit. Let these words feed you at your core so you can have the life you want and deserve.

Bach, David	*The Automatic Millionaire*
Burchard, Brendon	*Life's Golden Ticket*
	The Millionaire Messenger
Byrne, Rhonda	*The Secret*
Coelho, Paulo	*The Alchemist*
	The Aleph
Chopra, Deepak	*Perfect Health*
	The Seven Spiritual Laws of Success
Clason, George S.	*The Richest Man in Babylon*
David, Marc	*Nourishing Wisdom*
Dyer, Wayne	*The Power of Intention*
Ehrmann, Max	*Desiderata*
Gibran, Khalil	*The Prophet*
Gilbert, Elizabeth	*Eat, Pray, Love*
Hay, Louise	*You Can Heal Your Life*
Kiyosaki, Robert	*Rich Dad, Poor Dad*
	Cashflow Quadrant

Klemmer, Brian	*The Compassionate Samurai*
	If How To's Were Enough, We'd All Be Skinny, Rich, and Happy
Lad, Vasant	*The Science of Self-Healing*
Northrup, Christiane	*The Secret Pleasures of Menopause*
Pert, Candace	*Molecules of Emotion*
Rosenthal, Joshua	*Integrative Nutrition*
Roth, Geneen	*Women, Food, and God*
Weil, Andrew	*Eight Weeks to Optimum Health*
Williamson, Marianne	*A Course in Weight Loss*

Have a Juicy Day

Include juicy activities in your day so you turn your "To-Do's" into "Ta-DA's!"

What goes on your list?

Yoga in the morning	Read a favorite novel
Meditation	Play a game with kids
Walk by the water	Rent a movie
Leisurely breakfast	Write a blog post
Manicure/pedicure	Call your best friend

Now create your to-do list:

(To-DO) _____

(Juicy 1) _____

_____

_____

(Juicy 2) _____

_____

_____

(Juicy 3) _____

_____ (Ta-DA!)

Pleasure Play List
(Part 1)

Luxurious Self-Massage

Give yourself an aromatherapy self-massage. Use a luxurious massage oil like warm (melted) coconut oil, jojoba oil, grape seed oil, or almond oil. Choose essential oil of lavender for relaxation, jasmine and patchouli to prepare for a romantic evening, and eucalyptus and lemon to increase energy.

Allow at least 20-30 minutes for this pampering act of self-love. Take off all your clothes. Do this in the bathroom while standing on a towel. Light some candles, play some soft music, and make sure the room is warm so you don't get chilled.

Pour some oil into the palm of your hand. Rub your hands together to warm the oil and then slowly rub it into your scalp and all over your head. Use plenty of oil.

With just the oil on your hands, slowly and methodically massage your face and ears. Make sure you massage the ridge under your eyebrows, where the bridge of your nose meets the forehead, and your jaw line.

Now you can use as much oil as you want for the rest of the massage. Use downward strokes down the front of your body, rubbing in circles around all your joints. Use upward strokes up the back of your body (put oil on the backs of your hands to reach your back). Don't forget your buttocks, hips, and abdomen.

For greater nourishment and to get some Vitamin G (Gratitude) at the same time, as you massage each body part, thank it for supporting you and for all the things it does for you.

When you are finished, sit quietly for a few minutes (on a towel so you don't get oil everywhere), and feel the difference in your body. Take several deep breaths, and when you feel complete, take a long, warm shower, nourishing your body again with love and appreciation for all it has done for you.

Let the Dogs Out

Soak your feet in hot water for about 10 minutes. Practice deep breathing while your feet are soaking. Dry thoroughly with a soft towel, and begin to give yourself a slow, mindful foot rub. Pay attention to the space between each of your toes and the arch of your foot. When your foot is dry, rub in some peppermint lotion or cream. Paint your toes a crazy color.

Give Yourself a Facial

If you have some face and body products, bring a bunch of them out and treat yourself to the whole regimen: cleansing, exfoliation, toning or moisturizing mask, skin pH toner, brightening cream, eye cream, moisturizing lotion. Use the cleansing lotion/cream or exfoliant to massage your face and neck. While the mask is "setting," you can do that foot rub...

When All Else Fails...

Grab your favorite pillow, lie down on the floor in the sun, and take a cat nap (or a puppy nap).

Relax and Restore

Listen to a Guided Meditation CD.

Sit down and listen to a favorite CD with headphones on. Really listen to the words.

Set a timer for five minutes. Breathe deeply, in through your nose, out through your mouth. Think the word "so" on your inhale and the word "hum" on the exhale.

Have your child paint your toes.

Go outside, take your shoes off, and stand in the grass. Close your eyes and imagine you are a tree, with your roots going deep into the earth, and your body stretching high into the sky. Breathe deeply and tune into your senses. What do you hear, feel, touch, smell?

Walk in rhythm to your breath. On your inhale take four steps. On your exhale take four steps. As long as you are doing this meditation (fast or slow), keep your attention on your breath and keeping the counts even.

Pull out an old yearbook and reminisce.

Take an aromatherapy bath. After you draw your bath, add 3-5 drops of essential oils. Choose lavender for calming the mind, jasmine for cooling the body, and ginger and cinnamon for rejuvenation.

Values for Vibrancy

This list of values is a partial list. Only you know what goes on your list. Choose 10 that pop out at you. Then start noticing how you live your life and what you choose. By doing so, you will discover what is important to you and fills your heart and soul with vibrancy.

Abundance	Honor
Achievement	Independence
Adventure	Influencing others
Affection	Integrity
Arts	Knowledge
Boldness	Location
Commitment	Loyalty
Community	Order
Competition	Physical challenge
Contribution	Privacy
Control	Public service
Creativity	Recognition
Decisiveness	Religion
Effectiveness	Reputation
Efficiency	Security
Excitement	Self-respect
Fame	Serenity
Fast pace	Stability
Focus	Status
Freedom	Time freedom
Friendships	Tranquility
Growth	Trust
Having a family	Variety
Honesty	Wealth

Wellness Wheel

Directions: The eight sections in the Wellness Wheel represent facets of your life. With the center of the wheel as 1 and the outer edge as 10, rank your level of satisfaction with each life area (write the number by the label) and draw a line to create a new outer edge. The new perimeter of the circle represents the Wheel of Life.

How bumpy would the ride be if this were a real wheel? An additional perspective to consider is that you may be currently choosing to give one area of your life more emphasis in time and energy than another. Expect your wheel to reflect those decisions. Are you satisfied with your choices?

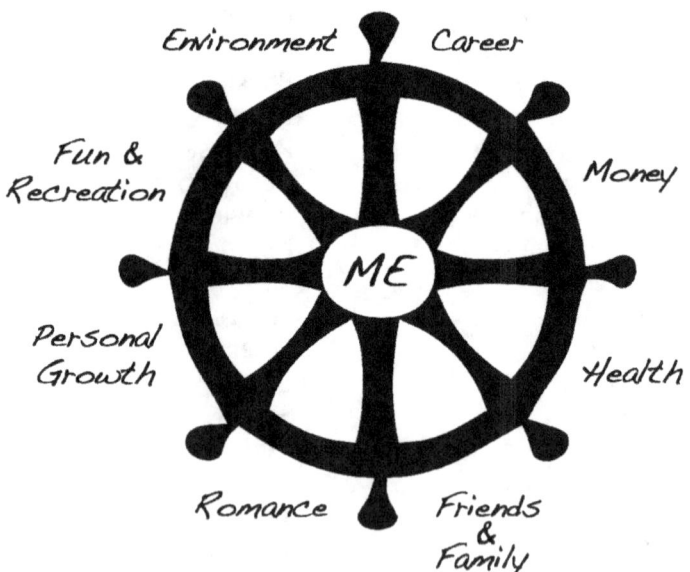

WORDS TO
NOURISH YOUR SOUL
Master Chefs'
Recipes for Success

Follow your bliss, and the Universe will open doors for you where there were only walls.

Joseph Campbell, *The Power of Myth*

You create your own universe as you go along.

Winston Churchill, as quoted in *The Secret*

Whether you think you can or you can't, either way you are right.

Henry Ford, as quoted in *The Secret*

It is impossible to live pleasurably without living wisely, well, and justly, and it is impossible to live wisely, well, and justly without living pleasurably.

Epicurus, as quoted in
The Slow Down Diet by Marc David

I am the bread of life. He who comes to me will never go hungry, and he who believes in me will never be thirsty.

Jesus of Nazareth, *The Bible*, John 6:35, NIV

There is no lack. There is more than enough. You are more than enough. Thus, there is an abundant supply of everything you need.

Brian Klemmer, *The Compassionate Samurai*

Eating a good meal with people you love streamlines the process of digestion and contributes to glowing health.

Christiane Northrup, M.D., *Women's Wisdom* perpetual calendar

Nourish the mind like you would your body. The mind cannot survive on junk food.

Jim Rohn, *The Treasury of Quotes by Jim Rohn*

To know you have enough is to be rich.

Tao Te Ching, 2009 wall calendar

Don't be reluctant to give of yourself generously. It's the mark of caring and compassion and personal greatness.

Brian Tracy, *The Treasury of Quotes by Brian Tracy*

You can rise above, stay in love, reach your goal, be happy in your soul. It's your attitude. If you think you can, you can.

Denis Waitley, *If You Think You Can, You Can* (song lyrics)

The body has a natural intelligence for creating and maintaining the perfect weight for you as long as the mind is aligned with its own perfection.

Marianne Williamson, *A Course in Weight Loss*

Pleasure Play List
(Part 2)

Singing and listening to uplifting music nourishes me deeply. I hope the lyrics to these songs make your heart sing.

Attitude

Ac-cent-tchu-ate the Positive (Aretha Franklin)

Blue Skies (Keepsake, Barbershop Quartet)

Don't Worry, Be Happy (Bobby McFerrin)

59th Street Bridge Song (Feeling Groovy) (Simon and Garfunkel)

Books

Paperback Writer (The Beatles)

Unwritten (Natasha Bedingfield)

Colors

The Lady in Red (Chris DeBurgh)

Tapestry (Carole King)

Diversity

Why Can't We be Friends (War)

Endorphins

Gonna Make You Sweat (Everybody Dance Now) (C+C Music Factory)

Friends and Family

House at Pooh Corner (Loggins and Messina)

Gratitude

I Thank You (Sam and Dave)

Holism

Dry Bones (Lennon Sisters)

Integration

Putting It Together (Barbra Streisand)

Juiciness

Don't Rain on My Parade (Barbra Streisand)

Kisses

Butterfly Kisses (Bob Carlisle)

Just Kiss Me (Harry Connick Jr.)

Love (Romantic)

For Once in My Life (Stevie Wonder)

Until I Met You (Manhattan Transfer)

Love (Love of Child)

With Arms Wide Open (Creed)

Baby, Baby (Amy Grant)

Love (Love of Self)

Hero (Mariah Carey)

Greatest Love of All (Whitney Houston)

Money

If You Had All the World and Its Gold (Growing Girls, Barbershop Quartet)

Nature

Rocky Mountain High (John Denver)

The Eagle and the Hawk (John Denver)

Oxygen

The Air That I Breathe (The Hollies)

Breathe (Faith Hill)

Pleasure

I Got You (I Feel Good) (James Brown)

Walkin' on Sunshine (Katrina and the Wave)

Quality

Wouldn't It Be Loverly (Julie Andrews)

Relaxation

The Lazy Song (Bruno Mars)

Sailing (Christopher Cross)

Simplicity

The Secret o' Life (James Taylor)

Simple Gifts (Yo-Yo Ma and Alison Krauss)

Simple Joys (from Pippin)

Time

A Cup of Coffee, a Sandwich, and You (Jack Buchanan and Gertrude Lawrence)

We've Got Tonight (Bob Seger)

Understanding

It's About Time (John Denver)

You've Got a Friend (Carole King)

Vibrancy

Live Like You Were Dyin' (Tim McGraw)

Xeriscape

Colors of the Wind (Vanessa Williams)

This Land Is Your Land (Peter, Paul, and Mary)

Yes!

Shout (Isley Brothers)

Zest for Life

Celebration (Kool and the Gang)

What a Wonderful World (Louis Armstrong)

You Make Me Feel So Young (Frank Sinatra)

ABOUT THE AUTHOR

Sally Galloway is a self-avowed natural health "geek" and an active food coach and foodie. For almost three decades, she has been teaching her clients and students how to nourish themselves. As a motivational speaker and wellness educator for corporations and retreats, Sally has been described as "funny," "dynamic," and "passionate."

Her professional alphabet soup includes MME (Master of Music Education), NCMT (Nationally Certified Massage Therapist), CHHC, AADP (Holistic Health Counselor, Certified by the American Association of Drugless Practitioners), CPCC (Certified Professional Co-Active Coach), GFI (Group Fitness Instructor), LWC (Licensed WellCoach), Ayurvedic Practitioner, and other morsels that occasionally appear on her plate.

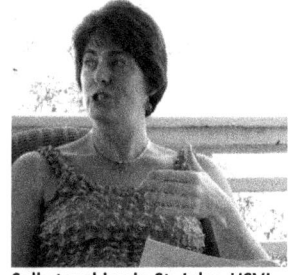

Sally teaching in St. John, USVI

You are invited to be a part of the blog community at *http://www.nutrition-counseling.com/spiritualfood,* and pull a chair up to the table to join one of her classes, webinars, or delicious retreats.